I0792121

ISBN: 9781674821382

101
Lifelong
Fitness
Tips and 'Secrets'

Compiled by

NoPaperPress staff

<u>101 Lifelong Fitness</u>

<u>Tips and 'Secrets'</u>

Compiled by the NoPaperPress™ staff

The following are offered to help you get physically fit in a healthy and effective manner. Use the tips that apply to you and that can best help you succeed. Good luck!

<u>Basic Fitness Tips & Secrets</u>

1) To get fit and stay fit, exercise regularly, do not smoke, practice good nutrition, maintain a proper weight level, and have periodic medical checkups.

2) Benefits of being fit: Lower blood pressure; a stronger and more efficient heart; supple and young arteries; a higher metabolic rate; larger more powerful muscles with more definition, and stronger bones.

3) When you're physically fit, you'll look and feel younger than your chronological age and you'll probably live longer too.

4) To prevent or delay the onset of type II diabetes, experts urge the overweight to lose weight and work out regularly.   Weight loss helps your body use insulin more efficiently, and exercise helps metabolize excess blood glucose.

5) You should have a medical exam, before starting a physical fitness program. This is especially important if you are overweight, if you have been inactive, if you have a history of medical problems, or if you are 40 or older.

6) Remember to discuss your physical fitness plan and your short-term and long-term goals with your doctor.

7) Before you start a physical fitness program you should know your current fitness level. Assessing your current level in areas such as aerobic (cardio) capacity, strength, flexibility, body-fat, will help you determine what you should emphasize and help you set realistic goals.

8) A good measure of your cardio-respiratory fitness, is the volume of oxygen per minute per kilogram of body weight (called VO2max) you can process during hard exercise.

9) A good self-assessment test for VO2max is the Rockport Walking Test. After walking a mile as rapidly as you can, you record your pulse and the time to complete the walk. You then convert your time and pulse into VO2max using formulae and a table in "Total Fitness – U.S. Edition" (by NoPaperPress.com).

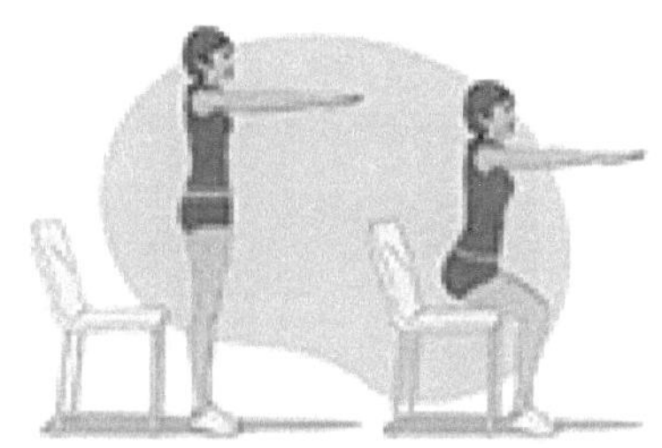

10) Self-assessment strength tests include the Push-up Test, the Sit-up Test, and the Squat Test. (For descriptions of the tests and to interpret your test results and see how fit you are, see "Total Fitness – U.S. Edition").

11) The standard self-assessment test for flexibility is the "Sit and Reach Test." (Again see "Total Fitness – U.S. Edition.")

12) Exercise physiologists consider the percentage of body fat compared to total body weight a critical measure of fitness, and contend, from the standpoint of good health, that men should have no more than 20 percent body fat and women no more than 23 percent body fat.

13) It's more practical to use Body Mass Index, or BMI, to determine what you should weigh. Your BMI is calculated by dividing your weight in kilograms by the square of your height in meters. (Again see "Total Fitness – U.S. Edition," by NoPaperPress.com for a convenient, easy-to-use chart).

14) Another important health parameter is your waist-to-hip ratio. Your risk for heart attack and stroke increase considerably for men with a ratio above 1.0 and for women with a ratio above 0.8. To calculate your ratio, measure your waist (at its narrowest section) and divide it by your hip (at its widest section).

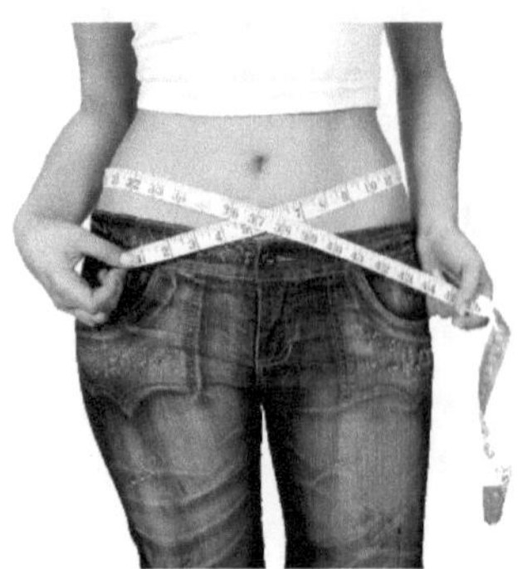

<u>**Basic Exercise Tips & Secrets**</u>

15) Muscle is active tissue, fat is not. The more muscle you have, the more calories you burn. Muscle uses a significant number of calories every day for repair and rebuilding giving your metabolism a boost even when you're resting. So make sure strengthening exercises (like weight lifting) are part of your workout.

16) Stay Busy. Most people will do anything to avoid work, housework, yard work, exercise, etc.   But any kind of work burns a lot more calories than just sitting. Whatever it is you are avoiding – just go and do it!

17) Consider anytime you have to lift, bend, reach, walk as an opportunity to burn additional calories and as an extension of your formal workout.

18) Get a good chart (like the one in Total Fitness - U.S. Edition) that lists how many calories are burned for different activities – depending on what you weigh.

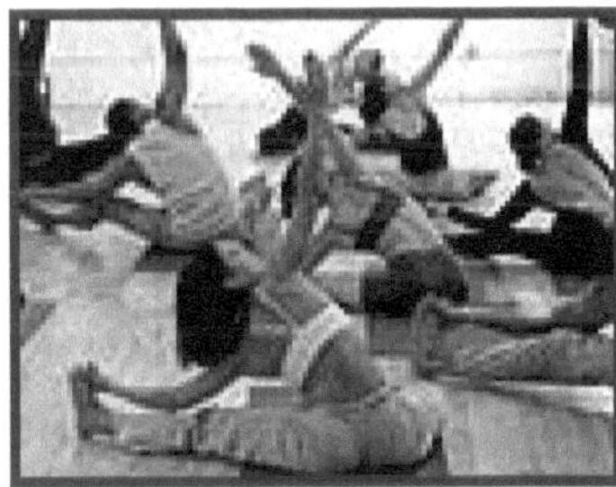

19) For any activity, the more you weigh the more calories you burn!

20) Engage in leisure activities such as dancing, bowling and gardening more often. They can be enjoyable and provide added exercise.

21) If you work at a desk, stand up and stretch two or three times a day, read standing up, etcetera.

22) If you've been inactive for some time, rather than starting with one of the more strenuous exercises, you should initially confine yourself to walking until you

can easily walk two miles at a brisk pace. When you reach this stage more strenuous exercises can be attempted if desired.

23) Some sports medicine physicians contend that if you are badly overweight you should limit your exercise to walking until you are less than 25 percent overweight.

24) An exercise buddy can make exercise more enjoyable and can help you get going and keep going on days when you might otherwise quit.

25) On the other hand, an exercise partner probably means that you now have the schedules of two busy people to contend with and plan around, which can at times actually hinder your workout.

26) You must be open to rearranging your priorities to fit exercise into your daily life.

27) To improve muscle tone and overall fitness, feel good and stay healthy, you should exercise at least five days per week, day after day, week after week, year after year – for as long as you are physically able.

28) Remember exercise key words: consistent, determined, steady, persistent, dogged, unswerving, gritty, single-minded. Consistent!

Walking Tips & Secrets

29) Walking is a wonderful exercise. It's an exercise you can do anywhere, that you can do well into your old age, that you can do outdoors or indoors, and that requires no special equipment other than a good comfortable pair of walking shoes. Whereas, joining and working out at a fitness center can be relatively expensive.

30)   Buy a pedometer and start walking. For the average person 2,100 steps amounts to walking about one mile. A Harvard study has shown that 8,000 to 10,000 step per day promotes weight loss.

31) Walk to burn calories and lose weight. You burn about 100 calories for each mile that you walk. Jogging burns about the same 100 calories per mile – but in a shorter time.

32) 160 lb person (man or woman) walking at 3.5 mph burns about 320 Calories in one hour.

33) not only helps you lose weight but also has many health benefits. So when you walk – don't saunter - walk briskly.

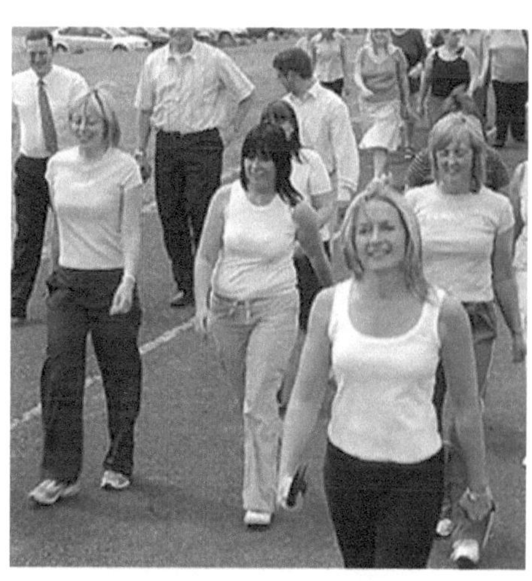

34) Look for opportunities to walk, such as walking to a local store rather than driving, walking the course if you play golf, and mowing your lawn.

35) For extra exercise, park within walking distance

of your destination and walk, and if you're healthy walk up stairs rather than taking an elevator or escalator.

36) For more exercise, take a brisk 15 minute walk around the mall before you start shopping.

37)   For life-long weight control take a vigorous 30 to 60 minute walk everyday! That's right – everyday. Make exercise a nonflexible top priority part of your life.

Cardio Tips & Secrets

38) Aerobic (cardio) exercises, such as jogging, swimming, cycling, brisk walking, skipping rope, and many others, are typically deep breathing and continuous, with rhythmic and repetitive contractions of your large muscle groups.

39) Most aerobic exercises have one thing in common: they make you work hard and require you to process a great deal of oxygen.

40) If you want to strengthen your heart and lungs, improve your aerobic capacity and burn a lot of calories select a vigorous aerobic activity such as jogging.

41) A classic aerobic exercise routine consists of a warm up, your main exercise, and a cool down period.

42) If you jog, always choose endurance over intensity; i.e., choose distance rather than speed, choose to jog longer rather than faster.

43) If you decide to exercise outdoors you should also have an alternate indoor activity, an activity you can fall back on in bad weather.

44) If you jog outside early in the morning before work, you may want to purchase a treadmill for use at home on days when it is either too hot, too cold or the weather is just bad.

45) Be aware that the pounding your body gets from jogging usually takes its toll over time. Many joggers have recurring, nagging injuries, particularly to their legs and feet.

46) If you start to suffer chronic injuries, try other high-intensity aerobic exercises for which your body might be better suited such as cycling, a rowing machine, etc.

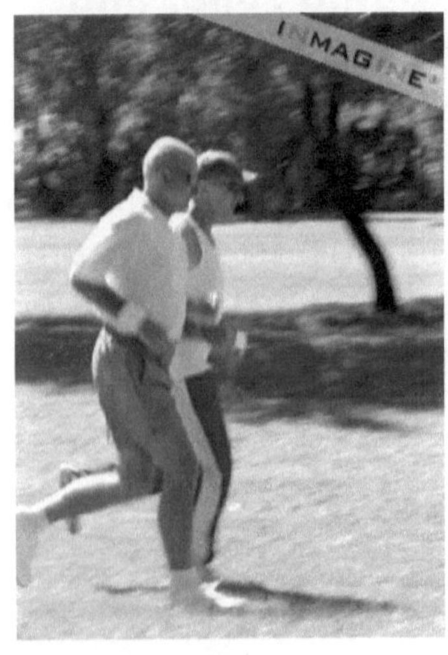

47) You if you cannot converse comfortably with a partner while you are walking briskly, jogging, cycling, etc. A feeling of having worked hard is fine, sweating is good, but not a feeling of undo fatigue.

48) Potentially serious problems are signaled if you experience any of the following during or after exercise: Symptoms include but are not limited to difficulty breathing; abnormal heart action such as irregular heart rhythm; pain or pressure in the middle of your chest; pain in an arm or your neck; dizziness, fainting or lightheadedness; severe exhaustion; sudden loss of coordination; or confusion. If you experience any of these symptoms, stop exercising immediately and get medical help.

49) Another definition of the beneficial yet safe aerobic exercise region is referred to as the "Target Training Zone," which is determined by monitoring your pulse. The idea is to raise your pulse through exercise to a specific range (the target training zone) and hold it there for an extended period to obtain a cardiovascular benefit.

50) The American College of Sports Medicine recommends an exercise heart rate of 60 to 90 percent of your maximum heart rate should be maintained for about 30 to 45 minutes three to five days per week to become reasonably fit.

51) To monitor the intensity of your exercise, you should occasionally stop during your workout and take your pulse immediately. (To find your pulse, quickly place the tips of two fingers on a carotid artery in your neck. Then count the beats for ten seconds and multiply by six.)

Hot Weather Tips & Secrets

52) The ideal exercise temperature range is about 40 to 85°F with a wind speed less than 15 mph.

53) When you engage in vigorous exercise, your body generates a great deal of heat. On hot humid summer days, your body temperature can rise from 98.6°F up to 101°F. (A body temperature of 105°F is life threatening.)

54) In hot weather, be guided by the Heat Index, or apparent temperature, which combines the effects of air (dry bulb) temperature and relative humidity.

**55) Before exercising outdoors in hot weather, check your local weather forecast. If the forecast does not incorporate the heat index, you can use the forecasted air temperature
and relative humidity to determine a heat index value using tables, such as those in "Total Fitness - U.S. Edition" by Vincent Antonetti, PhD - published by NoPaperPress.**

56) Exercising when the Heat Index is 90 to 105°F can result in muscle cramps and/or heat exhaustion. The much more dangerous heat stroke is possible when the Heat Index is over 105°F.

57) Unless you are relatively young and in very good physical condition, it's not a good idea to engage in vigorous outdoor exercise when the heat index is over 90°F.

58) Drinking water is important for good health, but it's even more important on hot days while you are exercising. During vigorous exercise, you can lose one to two quarts of water

per hour in sweat, so when you exercise it's essential
to use common sense and stay hydrated.

Cold Weather Tips & Secrets

59) Many people exercise outdoors at temperatures well below 40°F.   To an exerciser, cold weather is usually less dangerous than extremely hot weather to an exerciser – but definitely is not risk-free.

60) Very low ambient temperatures combined with the wind increase the amount of heat leaving your body. As the wind speed increases, the temperature of any exposed skin drops
even further.

61) In cold weather, be guided by the Wind Chill Temperature Index which is a measure of the relative discomfort due to combined cold temperature and wind.

62) Potentially serious consequences of very low wind-chill temperatures are frostbite, hypothermia and heart attack.

63) At wind-chill temperature of approximately 10°F exercising outdoors becomes increasingly uncomfortable. Even if you are an outdoor enthusiast, at this wind chill you may want to think about changing to an indoor exercise.

64) At a wind-chill temperature of approximately -17°F the risk of frostbite starts to increase.

65) Before exercising outdoors in cold weather, check your local weather forecast. It's not a good idea to exercise outdoors when the wind-chill temperature is below -20°F
because any exposed skin will freeze in about 10 minutes.

66) If you insist on working out in very hot or cold weather, always let someone know when and where you will be exercising and when you are planning to return.

Strength Tips & Secrets

67) Your body has approximately 650 muscles that account for more than half your body weight.

68) As you age you loose muscle mass, your bone density decreases and you lose strength. Exercises like weight lifting strengthen your muscles, bones and joints and also reduce your risk of developing osteoporosis.

69) If you want to become physically stronger choose one of the strength-building exercises such as weight lifting.

70) Because strengthening exercises work a muscle until it's fatigued, take a day off between strength workouts for your muscles to recover, repair and rebuild.

71) in a bedroom, basement, garage, or attic. A set of variable (adjustable) weight dumbbells and a small weight bench don't take up much room and are all you need for a home-based gym.

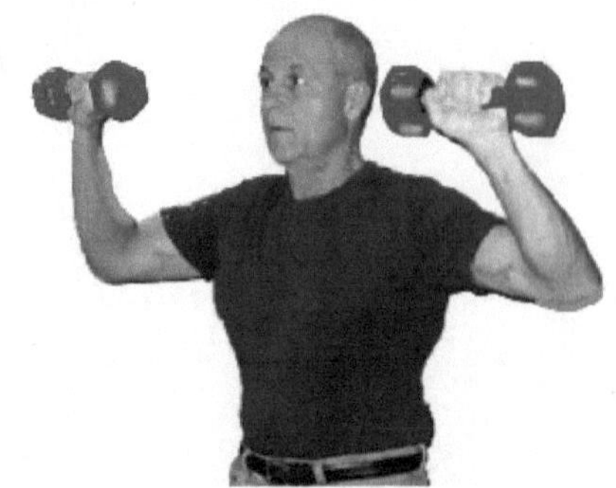

72) Working out at home has some significant advantages. Your workout takes less time because you don't have to drive back and forth to a fitness facility; and you have the flexibility of dividing your workout into small time segments to fit your day, and working out at home is less expensive.

73) Bear in mind, knowledge and the discipline to workout regularly are far more important than fancy equipment.

74) When you start weight training, rather than purchase an entire set of weights, buy just enough dumbbell weight so that you can do a military press five times.

75) Never hold your breath during weight training. This can cause your blood pressure to get dangerously high. Rather, breathe naturally and try to exhale during a lift.

76) If you only miss working out for a day or two, you can just pick up where you left off as if nothing happened. If you miss a week or more, you probably have lost some of your fitness gains and might have to resume at a somewhat lower exercising-intensity level. Listen to your body.

77) A common weight-loss fallacy is that you can lose abdominal fat by working your abdominal muscles. This is based on the incorrect belief that fat is eliminated from a particular part of your body if you engage the muscles underneath that layer of fat. No such luck.

78) To determine your frame size, circle your wrist with your thumb and third finger. If the tips of your fingers overlap, you have a small frame. If they just touch you are medium, and if they don't touch you have a large frame.

Injury Avoidance Tips & Secrets

79) Avoid injury by building up exercise intensity gradually over many weeks, months.

80) Avoid injury by waiting two hours after a meal before you start exercising.

81) Avoid injury by waiting 30 minutes after exercising before you eat.

82) Avoid injury by using safety and protective equipment as appropriate, such as helmet when you bicycle, and goggles when you play handball, squash or racquetball.

83) Avoid injury by warming up and cooling down slowly.

84) Avoid injury by not increasing the difficulty of any activity (e.g., your walking or jogging distance, the amount of weight you lift) by more than 10 percent per week.

85) Avoid injury by jogging on softer surfaces such as a level grass field, a dirt path, or a running track.

86) Many minor leg injuries of the muscles and joints can be treated using the well-known R.I.C.E. method, i.e., rest, ice, compression, elevation.

87) Attend an orientation session before you use any unfamiliar exercise equipment. Otherwise, read the operating instructions carefully.

<u>**Nutrition Tips & Secrets**</u>

88) An understanding of nutrition is not only vital for good health but also helps you control your weight in the long term.

89) The diet of most Americans is not very healthy. We consume too many calories and too much saturated fat, trans fat, cholesterol, added sugars and salt.

90) Drink lots of water – about 8 glasses per day. Try adding a slice of lemon to make it more interesting. Often, when you think you're hungry, you're just thirsty. So, next time you reach for a snack, drink some water first and see if that does it for you.

91) Know your daily caloric allowance whether you are trying to maintain your weight or are on a reducing diet. (Again see "Total Fitness - U.S. Edition" by NoPaperPress where you can determine your daily caloric allowance using unique Weight Maintenance tables.)

92) Eat a variety of foods within your caloric allowance, and use the USDA Pyramid to shape your eating patterns. Try to eat the recommended amount from each food group.

93) Do not eat foods containing partially-hydrogenated vegetable oil because they are high in trans fats. This includes commercially prepared baked goods, snack foods, and processed foods, including most fast foods.

94) Limit your intake of saturated fats. Eat meat less often and fish and poultry more often, and use fat-free or low-fat milk and milk products.

95) When possible, and
natural foods and whole-grain
products. Avoid chemical
preservatives and additives,
artificial and imitation foods,
refined and processed foods,
and foods that are comprised
of "nutritionally-empty
calories."

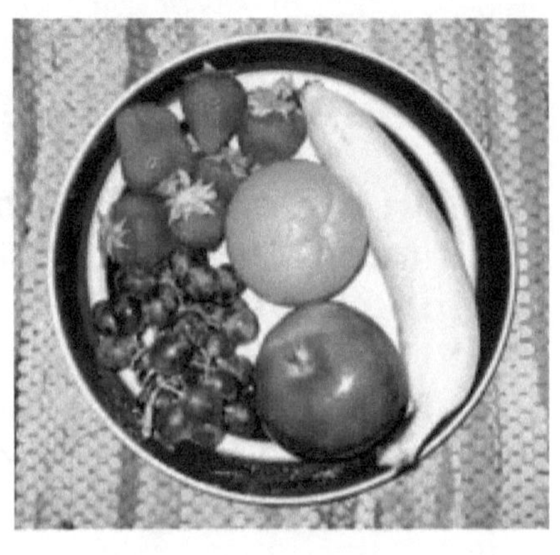

96) Fiber is an important part
of a healthy diet. According to the Harvard University
School of Public Health, adequate fiber intake reduces
your risk of developing various conditions, including
heart disease, diabetes, diverticular disease, and
constipation.

97)   When you eat fiber, it simply passes straight
through, untouched by but aiding your digestive
system. Zero calories absorbed!

98) Adults should get a least 20 to 35 grams of dietary
fiber per day. The best sources are fresh fruits and
vegetables, nuts and legumes, and whole-grain foods.

99) Most Americans consume too much sodium. The
U.S. Department of Agriculture Dietary Guidelines
recommend that healthy adults limit sodium intake to
2,400 mg per day. (Note one level teaspoon of salt
contains about 2,300 mg of sodium.)

100) Sugar should be used sparingly by people with
low calorie needs and in moderation by most other
healthy adults.

101) Contrary to what many believe, the latest
scientific evidence indicates adult-onset diabetes
occurs most often in those who are overweight.

<u>**Bonus Tips & Secrets**</u> (Nutrition continued)

102) Wine and beer contain a small amount of nutrients and micronutrients, but other alcoholic beverages, such as whiskey, vodka and gin consist of nothing but "nutritionally-empty calories."

103) Caffeine should be used in moderation. Caffeine is found in coffee, tea, some soft drinks and foods that contain cocoa. It is also in some drugs such as cold remedies and in medicine sold over the counter to relieve headaches.

104) The majority of exercise physiologists feel that sports drinks are unnecessary for most people, and that plain water, along with the salt in the food we eat, are all that is needed to replenish the water and sodium lost during <u>moderate</u> exercise.

105) Before you buy, read and understand the labels on food packages.

106) "Eat Slowly." This is especially vital when you're trying to lose weight. If you're someone who eats fast, you're not giving yourself a chance to feel full. While everyone else is still eating, you either sit and pick, or you have seconds, taking in extra calories you could avoid if you would just slow down.

<u>**Bonus Tips & Secrets**</u> (Weight Control)

107) It's a lot easier to eat 1,000 Calories than it is to burn 1,000 Calories by exercising. So a stroll after dinner won't offset the calories you ingest eating a big meal.

108)   Understand that the only sure way to slim down for keeps is to eat less and exercise more. There are no safe short cuts or miracle methods for taking off weight.

109) Successful weight loss and subsequent weight maintenance requires knowledge, desire and discipline. Avoid the latest fad diets. Instead, take the time to develop a true understanding of weight control and then change your eating and activity habits accordingly.

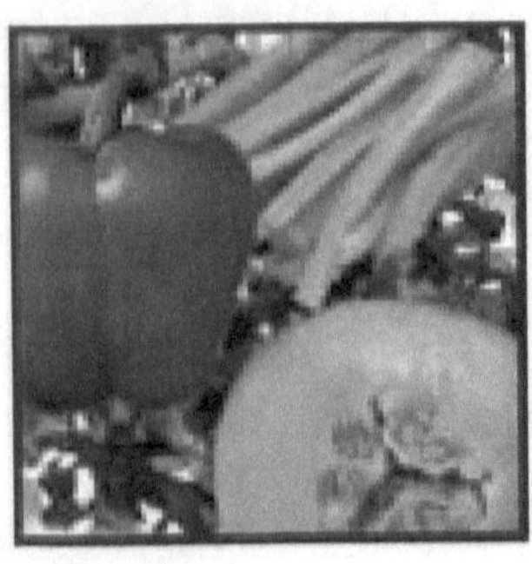

110) Consistently choose healthy foods, avoid harmful foods and large portions and exercise regularly. Nothing else will work over the long haul.

111) Experts agree that whether you are trying to lose weight or just maintain your weight, it's calories that count.   In theory it doesn't matter what foods the calories are from – to lose weight eat fewer calories than you burn.

112) Weight loss occurs when your food energy intake is less than the total energy you expend. This difference in calories is referred to as your calorie deficit.

113) How much weight you lose depends on the magnitude of your calorie deficit. To lose one pound requires a deficit of approximately 3,500 Calories.

114) If you are overweight start on a weight loss diet now because it will only become more difficult to lose weight as you get older.

115) Inevitably, everyone on a diet hits a exasperating weight-loss plateau. The only way to bust through the plateau is to reduce your calorie intake and/or to step up your exercise intensity.

116) Slow weight loss is healthier, is more likely to be permanent, and is easier to sustain over the long haul. So when it comes to weight loss, don't be in a hurry!

118) A very important weight-profile parameter is your waist-to-hip ratio. Health risks for heart attack and stroke increase considerably for men with a ratio above 1.0 and for women with a ratio above 0.8. To calculate your ratio, measure your waist size (at its narrowest circumference) and divide it by your hip size (at its widest section).

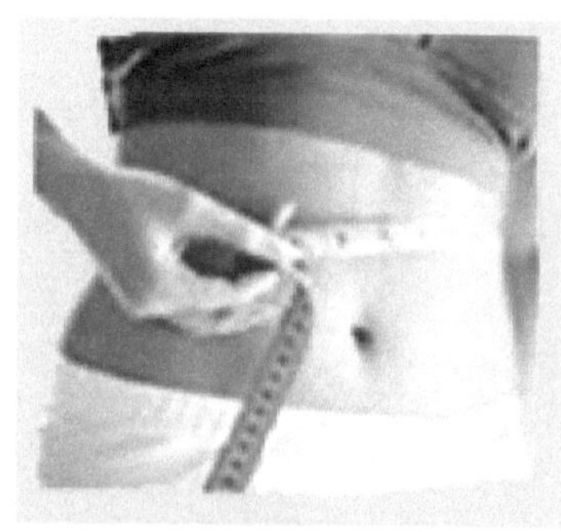

117) The general weight-loss rule is "last on first off." When you lose weight, it normally it will come off in the reverse order of where you gained it.   And there is not much you can do about that. There is no food, no exercise, no magic pill that will cause your body to lose fat in one place rather than another.

<u>Bonus Tips & Secrets</u> (Miscellaneous)

119)   Take a daily multi-vitamin/mineral supplement. This is important when you're on a diet – as a kind of insurance policy.

120) Keep a daily fitness log to record your progress. For some people it really works wonders.

121)   To get and stay fit and help control your weight, walk everyday and work out with dumbbells for twenty minutes two or three times a week. That's all most people need.

122) Finally, get a scientifically sound and effective weight control book to help you loss weight in a safe and healthy manner. Consider NoPaperPress, with its extensive line of weight control, nutrition and exercise eBooks written by experts for sensible adults

<u>NoPaperPress eBooks and Paperbacks</u>

100-Day Super Diet-1200 Cal*
100-Day Super Diet-1500 Cal*
100-Day No-Cooking Diet-1200 Cal*
100-Day No-Cooking Diet-1500 Cal*
90-Day Smart Diet-1200 Cal*
90-Day Smart Diet-1500 Cal*
90-Day No-Cooking Diet - 1200 Cal*
90-Day No-Cooking Diet - 1500 Cal*
90-Day Perfect Diet - 1200 Cal*
90-Day Perfect Diet - 1500 Cal*
60-Day Perfect Diet-1200 Cal*
60-Day Perfect Diet-1500 Cal*
50-Day Flex Diet-1200 Cal*
50-Day Flex Diet-1500 Cal*
30-Day Quick Diet - Women*
30-Day Quick Diet for Men*
30-Day No-Cooking Diet*
30-Day Diet for Women - Metric*
30-Day Diet for Men - Metric*
25 Day Easy Diet-1200 Cal*
25 Day Easy Diet-1500 Cal*
25-Day No-Cooking Diet
10-Day Express Diet
10-Day No-Cooking Diet*
7-Day Diet for Women*
7-Day Diet for Men*
7-Day No-Cooking Diets*
90-Day Gluten-Free Diet-1200 Cal*
90-Day Gluten-Free Diet-1500 Cal*
30-Day Gluten-Free Quick Diet*
30-Day Gluten-Free No-Cooking Diet*
7-Day Diet for Women - Metric*
7-Day Diet for Men - Metric
7-Day Gluten-Free Express Diet*
7-Day Gluten-Free No-Cooking Diet*
90-Day Vegetarian Diet-1200 Cal*
90-Day Vegetarian Diet-1500 Cal*
30-Day Vegetarian Diet*
7-Day Vegetarian Diet*
Weight Loss for Women*
Weight Loss for Women - Metric
Weight Loss for Women - UK
Weight Loss for Men*
Maximum Weight Loss - 1200 Cal*
Maximum Weight Loss - 1500 Cal*

Weight Loss for Men - Metric*
Maximum Weight Loss- 1200 Cal*
Maximum Weight Loss- 1500 Cal*
Weight Control - U.S. Edition*
Weight Control - Metric. Edition
Professional Weight Control Women - U.S.
Professional Weight Control Women - Metric
Professional Weight Control Men - U.S.
Professional Weight Control Men - Metric
Weight Maintenance - U.S. Ed*
Weight Maintenance - Metric. Ed*
Weight Maintenance - UK Ed
Weight Loss for Senior Men*
Weight Loss for Senior Women*
Eat Smart - U.S. Edition*
Eat Smart - Metric Edition
30-Day Mediterranean Diet
Exercise Smart - U.S. Edition*
Exercise Smart - Metric Edition
Exercise Smart - UK Edition*
Total Fitness - U.S. Edition
Total Fitness - Metric Edition
Total Fitness - UK Edition
Total Fitness for Women-U.S. Ed*
Total Fitness for Women - Metric
Total Fitness for Women - UK Ed
Total Fitness for Men - U.S. Ed*
Total Fitness for Men- Metric Ed*
Total Fitness for Men - UK Ed
Senior Fitness - U.S. Edition*
Senior Fitness - Metric Edition*
Senior Fitness - UK Edition*
Computer Diet - U.S. Edition*
Computer Diet - Metric Ed*
Reliable Weight Loss - U.S. Ed
101 Weight Loss Tips*
101 Healthy Eating Tips*
101 Lifelong Fitness Tips*
101 Weight Maintenance Tips
101 Weight Loss Recipes
101 GF Weight Loss Recipes
101 Veggie Weight Loss Recipes*
30-Day Mediterranean Diet*
90-Day Mediterranean Diet - 1200 Cal*
90-Day Mediterranean Diet - 1500 Cal*

* These titles are available as both ebooks and paperbacks. Our ebooks are sold by Amazon, Apple, Google, Barnes & Noble and Kobo, but our paperbacks are only sold by Amazon.

Disclaimer

This work offers general Nutrition, weight control and exercise information. It is not a medical manual and the authors do not claim to be medically qualified. The material in this book is not intended to be a substitute for medical counseling. Everyone should have a medical checkup before beginning a weight control, or exercise program. Moreover, the physician conducting the medical exam should be made aware of and should approve the specific weight control or exercise program planned. Additionally, while the authors and publisher have made every effort to ensure the accuracy of the information in this book, they make no representations or warranties regarding its accuracy or completeness. Further, neither the authors nor publisher assume liability for any medical problems that might result from applying the methods in this book, or for any loss of profit, or any other commercial damages, including but not limited to special, incidental, consequential or other damages, and any such liability is hereby expressly disclaimed.